THE WHEAT BELLY CURE

DISCOVER 10 COMMON HEALTH PROBLEMS CURED BY ADOPTING A WHEAT FREE DIET

I0420900

CHARLOTTE MOYER

Receive my next book for free!
Exclusive promotions, updates and newsletters
Join my Book Club Now

TABLE OF CONTENTS

CONCLUSION

ABOUT THE AUTHOR

OTHER BOOKS BY AUTHOR

WELCOME

Thank you for purchasing this book, *'The Wheat Belly Cure: Discover 10 Common Health Problems cured by Adopting a Wheat Free Lifestyle".*

Wheat and other grains are all-present in the Western diet. From supposedly 'healthy' home cooked meals to processed food and even most common sauces and condiments, wheat is everywhere.

However, our constant consumption of wheat and other grains is playing havoc with our bodies and well being. Not only does wheat cause us to gain weight, but it is also responsible for many common health ailments such as fatigue, acne and more. If you constantly find yourself bugged by a consistent and but undiagnosed health problem, cutting out the wheat and grains in our diet might be the only antidote you need.

This book provides the insight and science behind the increasingly popular wheat belly diet. In particular, learn about 10 common health problems and how they can all be caused by the presence of wheat and other grains in your diet.

Let's get started!

Charlotte Moyer

PS...Don't forget to join my Book Club

INTRODUCTION

The average person in the west quietly suffers from a range of mild health ailments. It may be the case that they struggle to concentrate clearly, or that they feel tired all the time. They may have persistent and stubborn acne that refuses to go away or suffer from migraines, seemingly without cause.

These maladies and many others often lack the severity to justify that trip down the doctor, or even to be recognized for an official diagnosis. Nonetheless, they are very real and influential in the lives of millions of people every day. In the face of large, life-threatening illness, these little issues may seem trivial and other people may fail to sympathize. Yet, when suffering from constant tiredness or weird unexplained allergic symptom, it is hard to live and enjoy life to the fullest.

Fortunately, there is a potential solution in sight; the wheat belly diet. The wheat belly diet advocates a shift in our dietary patterns; transitioning away from wheat, wheat products and sauces as well as other grains such as barley, rye and even rice. Instead, the wheat belly dieter enjoys a healthier array of foods; nuts, seeds, oils, meats, fish, vegetables, pulses and fruits.

In this book learn about all the benefits of embracing the wheat belly diet, grounded in a scientific and factual basis. In particular, this book will deal with the following 10 health issues commonly faced by many individuals following a modern western diet:

- Inflammation & Unexplained Allergies
- Acne
- Cholesterol & High Blood Pressure
- Fatigue & Energy levels, High Blood Sugar
- Obesity & Weight Gain
- Wrinkles & Aging
- Bloating, Constipation
- Brain fog and poor concentration
- Migraine relief
- Asthma and breathing problems

Learn how your brain fog may be due to a lack of fatty acids in your diet, or how acne may result from the relationship between wheat, insulin and bacteria and much more. If you suffer, or know someone who suffers from any of these problems, do not suffer in silence any more. Try the wheat belly diet; it may be the cure you are looking for.

UNDERSTANDING THE WHEAT BELLY CURE

Before you learn about the health benefits of the wheat belly diet, you may wish to know a little more about the diet itself and its key tenets. This chapter aims to teach you the basic premises of the wheat belly diet and why you should consider it superior to your current eating regime.

To put it simply, the wheat belly diet advocates a low-carbohydrate diet that avoids the carbohydrate sources popular in the western diet. These carbohydrates are noted to play havoc on our blood sugar levels affecting almost every aspect of our health.

The wheat belly diet is often adopted as a weight loss measure and tens of thousands of people have successfully shed the pounds by faithfully avoiding wheat and other problematic grains. The wheat-free diet, compared to many other weight loss diets is especially easy to maintain and rewarding to stick to because it is not a calorie controlled diet like almost every other weight loss diet out there; it just politely asks you to cut the wheat and other carbohydrates out of your diet and reap the rewards. You can eat however much you want, although most people find that their appetite becomes much more manageable by following the wheat belly diet and they eat less without any effort whatsoever.

Above and beyond the weight loss benefits of the wheat belly diet however, are also the health benefits as briefly explained in the introduction and explored in the rest of this book. Even if you are comfortable with your current size and shape, chances are the wheat belly diet and its much healthier diet will benefit you in some form. Whether you banish the brain fog or alleviate your allergies, a wheat-free diet can help you.

There are many other resources dedicated to the benefits of the wheat belly diet. However, essentially the entire diet breaks down into these three rules:

Avoid these foods:

Breakfast cereals

Noodles

Pasta

Bagels

Bread

Muffins

Pancakes

Waffles

Donuts

Crackers

Oats

Bran/ Bran Products

Cornstarch

Sauces/Gravies with starch

Chips

Tortillas

Soft Drinks

Candy

Ice Cream

Eat limited quantities of the following:

Fruit

Fruit Juice

Milk

Cheese

Cottage Cheese

Yogurt

Sweet Potato

Legumes

White Rice

Brown Rice

Soy Sauce

Dark Chocolate

Eat however much you want:

Vegetables

Almonds

Walnuts

Hazelnuts

Brazil Nuts

Cashews

Pumpkin seeds

Sunflower Seeds

Olive Oil

Flaxseed oil

Avocado

Walnut

Red meats

Tea

Coffee

Water

With this established, read the following chapter and to discover the fantastic rewards and advantages of following the wheat belly diet.

10 Common Health Problems Cured by a Wheat Belly Diet

Fatigue, Low Energy Levels & High Blood Sugar

You may have heard the term 'blood sugar' before, but many people are unaware of the vast importance and health implications associated with this aspect of our lives and diet.

Blood sugar refers to the concentration of glucose (sugar) in your blood. Glucose is the fuel your body uses for energy for nearly all metabolic functions such as the movement of your muscles and the activity in your brain. Your body requires a constant supply of glucose in the blood, if there is too little (hypoglycemia) your body cannot function but if there is too much sugar (hyperglycemia), severe health complications arise.

Owing to this, a healthy normal functioning human body has an entire system of chemicals and hormones that control and regulate the body's level of blood sugar. For example, you may be aware of insulin, which causes the body to transform excess blood sugar into fat (which we will talk about later).

However, these regulatory body systems can be compromised by a consistently poor diet and obesity leading to degenerative diseases as well as many other issues.

The most well-known disease to arise from the body's failure to control blood sugar is diabetes. In particular, type 2 diabetes occurs when due to long-term hyperglycemia caused by excess sugar or alcohol intake in the diet over many years. This causes the pancreas, which produces insulin, to become impaired. Levels of insulin in the body drops and the body also becomes insulin-resistant (insulin becomes less effective). As a result, high blood sugar levels are no longer moderated and the body starts to go haywire due to all the excess sugar in the system; heart disease, kidney failure, lower life expectancy and even amputation of the limbs (as well as many other devastating conditions) can all be caused by hyperglycemia.

Now you may be wondering how blood sugar is related to the wheat belly diet. The wheat belly diet prevents hyperglycemia and results in healthy levels of blood sugar. This prevents the occurrence of type 2 diabetes and all of the various health issues that arise with it.

Blood sugar levels are raised when the components of food you consume are broken down in the stomach and small intestine into glucose then released into the blood. Unlike other components of food, such as fiber, protein and fat, molecules such carbohydrates and sugars are broken down into glucose quicker than their peers. This causes more sugar to be released into the blood at once and blood sugar levels to spike.

Moreover, consistent and unhealthy consumption of these carbohydrates produces regular hyperglycemia and type 2 diabetes. Therefore, by embracing the wheat belly diet which is low in wheat, grains and other carbohydrates that produce worrisome blood sugar spikes, you can prevent hyperglycemia entirely.

Above and beyond severe and diagnosed conditions, the effects of these blood sugar spikes can cause low energy levels and fatigue. As formerly mentioned, your body needs glucose to function normally and healthily. However, when we consume foods that cause our blood sugar to spike, we only provide our bodies with glucose during that small duration when the blood sugar is spiking. After our blood sugar levels have crashed we are left with an energy deficit as our blood sugar levels become low. The result is a feeling of tiredness and a lack of energy to accomplish things.

The solution, however, is simple; consume foods that are broken down and release sugar into the blood slowly. As sugar is consistent and gradually released into the bloodstream, energy levels remain consistent and fatigue does not arise. Likewise, the harmful effects of hyperglycemia do not occur. This is what the wheat belly diet advocates; a diet high in fish, nuts, oils, seeds, meat, fruits and vegetables – foods which do not spike our blood sugar.

As a final parting note on this section, be aware that health issues due to hyperglycemia arise due to persistent abuse of our body's blood sugar. That solitary donut or piece of cake will not cause your body any harm; but a continual diet with regular consumption of donuts or cake will cause your body to suffer immensely. Use common sense and apply the rules of the wheat belly diet logically.

INFLAMMATION AND AUTO-IMMUNE RESPONSE

It is widespread knowledge that numerous people suffer from celiac disease and diagnosed wheat allergies. These people, upon consuming wheat, suffer violent and dangerous bodily symptoms, which can be life threatening. However, fewer people are aware of wheat intolerance, a milder condition than celiac disease or wheat allergy, but no less real. In addition to this, the adverse well being of wheat consumption in general and the subtle, but notable negative health impact wheat can leave on the general population.

If you find your skin displaying any of the signs of inflammation; redness, soreness, itchiness, swells or puffiness, the wheat and grains in your diet could be the cause. Often blotchy, red skin is taken as a sign of aging or a lack of exercise, but rash-like red skin across any region in the body may be your body's reaction to wheat and grains in your system.

Even more worrisome, many of these inflammatory symptoms can lead to other complications. If you find yourself with unexplained issues, such as joint pain, these could be caused by the retention of water producing pressure and strain around the ligaments and joints.

Often, one of the areas most affected by wheat consumption is the face, which becomes puffy and swollen due to inflammation. Even without losing weight, people who cut wheat from their diet may look slimmer and healthier as their face looses the swelling that seems as if it were excess weight.

Likewise, many individuals also suffer from swelling and inflammation around the feet and ankles making walking, running or even sitting in certain positions much more uncomfortable. Prolonged inflammation around these areas can also lead to skin conditions and rashes, which can become infected.

Furthermore, wheat may also be culpable for fever-like symptoms frequently attributed to hay fever and other allergies, such as sneezing, watery eyes, blocked sinuses and other similar problems.

Wheat contains a cocktail of proteins called gliadin. Gliadin is a complex and plant based protein that the human body struggles to digest and break-down. Above and beyond this, the body struggles to recognize gliadin as a protein molecule, as opposed to any other type of molecule, such as a carbohydrate or even a pathogen. Owing to this, when you consume gliadin, your body's immune system reacts as if a pathogen had just entered your system. Your body's reaction to pathogens is to trigger various bodily responses such as swelling of the skin and sneezing (responses you might recognize from other allergies).

Likewise, this swelling and inflammation does not have to be localized in a specific area. In fact, your immune systems response to a continual consumption of gliadin can cause your entire body to retain excess water, causing you to look and feel fatter than you actually are.

Obesity & Weight Gain

Obesity is an epidemic but no-one in the west seems to have the vaccine. We know that from a very rudimental perspective, weight gain is caused by consuming more calories than you expend. Yet this knowledge clearly isn't helping the populous, who not only pile on the pounds faster than ever before in the history of humankind, but fail to lose this weight once they have gained it.

Even amongst those of us who are not overweight, most of us have unhealthy relationships with our bodies and with our food. We may be a little soft around the edges without those fickle BMI machines telling us that we are overweight, or we may always feel like we are hungry or ravenous but never satiated by the foods we eat. With our diets and societal pressures being the way they are, there is always the constant threat and undertone that if you slip and let your eating habits get out of sync for just a few weeks or a month or two, you can start a downhill spiral and never come back.

However, the wheat belly diet advocates a new position on weight loss; cut out the wheat, grains and other problematic calorie sources in your diet and you will lose weight. This weight loss is caused by the several advantageous effects of the wheat belly diet; firstly, your body loses excess water that is has been retaining due to the masses of carbohydrates you have been eating. The overall result of this is a rapid weight loss over a short period of time as your body quickly dumps all this unnecessary water from your system.

The second effect, however, is lowered appetite. This advantage is actually caused by two separate factors, both related to the wheat belly diet. By taking it upon yourself to stick to the wheat belly diet, you consume more foods which produce greater levels of satiation. Foods which contain greater amounts of fiber, fat or protein and low amounts of carbohydrates tend to be digested slower in the stomach and the small intestine. Owing to the stomach being fuller with food for longer, less appetite signals are produced by the nervous system, which automatically triggers when the stomach starts to become empty.

Likewise, as many common foods that are high in carbohydrates also tend to be high in calories, people who still eat wheat and other grains struggle to consume a quantity of these foods which is large enough to produce satiation, but small enough to be within an acceptable range of calories. However, by eating the wheat belly diet, you can eat a greater amount of vegetables and fruit, resulting in a greater raw quantity of food consumed and less hunger.

The second influence of the wheat belly diet on appetite is how the diet affects blood sugar. In addition to how full our stomachs are, our bodies also produce hunger signals when our blood sugar runs too low. The sugar in our blood provides the necessary energy for our muscles and brain to keep functioning; when this level runs too low, our body tells us that we need to eat to increase our blood sugar levels.

However, wheat, grains and other problematic carbohydrate sources all cause our blood sugar levels to spike and fall quickly and dramatically. As these carbohydrates are easily digested and naturally high in sugar, our blood sugar level rises rapidly post-consumption. However, because all this blood sugar has been released into the body rapidly, as opposed to gradually over time, our blood sugar subsequently collapses an hour or two post-consumption.

The ultimate product of this blood sugar collapse, as previously described, is our body becomes desperate for more sugar and produces hunger signals. Hunger signals encourage us to eat even more and thus exceed our designated amount of calories we can eat per day and result in weight-gin. Therefore, wheat, grains and other carbohydrates are directly responsible for excessive calorie intake in many individuals and weight gain due to their negative influence on our appetite levels.

In addition to this, wheat, grains and other particular sources of carbohydrates may cause weight-gain by the method in which they are processed by the body. As formerly explained, these carbohydrate sources produce spikes in the body's blood sugar. However, our body, when faced with more energy than it requires (in the form of sugar) can store and transform this sugar into fat. Therefore when our blood sugar is particularly high, our body starts to partition some of this sugar into fat, increasing our weight.

To conclude this sub-section, not only do wheat, grains and other problematic carbohydrate sources cause us to have higher appetites but they also produce weight gain by how the body deals with the high blood sugar levels they produce. The effect of this is a two-fold attack on our bodies, causing us to both eat more and store more of the energy we eat as fat; it is no wonder then, with the prevalence of these carbohydrates in our diet that obesity is such a problem.

Early Aging

We all want to get rid of the wrinkles and keep that youthful vigor we maintained during our younger years. Some people seem to exist that grow and age gracefully; not only looking fresher and younger than they actually are, but also maintaining an unusual bodily health. These people walk with a spring in their step, without any of the tiresome and frequent body pains associated with entering our geriatric years.

The secret to preventing early aging is to realize that how we visibly and internally age is influenced by a myriad of factors, many of which are under your control. You do not have to resign yourself to looking like a centenarian once you are middle-aged, citing factors such as genetics as the cause of your appearance. Even if you are fortunate enough to still be young right now, you too will inevitably age; it is best to heed the following advice and take some preventative action.

One of the greatest causes of early aging is *advanced glycation end products (AGE's)*. These are certain molecules and compounds found within our cells which are known to contribute and increase susceptibility to degenerative and problematic health conditions, such as Diabetes, Alzheimer's disease and Atherosclerosis. As we age, the amount of advanced glycation end products found within our body increases; higher rates are detected in the skin and vital organs such as the kidneys, thus partially explaining the correlation between increased age and greater rates of degenerative disease.

Advanced glycation end products, commonly abbreviated in nutrition science and biology to AGE's are long complex glucose-protein molecules that accumulate in the bodily system. These molecules cannot be removed and they cause chaos with most of our bodies necessary functions; they clog the liver and the kidney, preventing the filtering of bodily waste and toxins. They also accumulate in the veins, arteries and joints, increasing blood pressure as well as making the joints and tendons less supple and more inflexible. AGE's are even claimed to influence the brain and it's biochemistry, causing the ever-present but hard-to-diagnose 'brain fog' and poor concentration that many of us seem to suffer with as we grow older.

However, as previously implied, advanced glycation end products are produced not only be natural aging, but also by controllable factors. One of these factors is persistently high blood glucose and sugar intake. As AGE's are glucose-protein molecules, their creation by the body directly increases with high blood sugar and glucose intake; an effect caused by wheat and grains.

You certainly cannot prevent aging altogether; it is inevitable that AGE's will gradually increase within your body. However, by cutting down on wheat, grains and other problematic carbohydrate sources, you can slow down the rate at which AGE's produced, keeping your youth and health present for longer.

ACNE

Acne is a skin condition that results in whiteheads, blackheads and deeper pus-filled pustules which commonly occur across the face, chest or back. Acne is generally associated with hormone and chemical changes during puberty, and the overwhelming majority of teenagers in the west are affected by the condition to varying degrees of intensity. However, acne can is also common for many people up to the age of thirty, and it can potentially affect people of all ages.

Although acne is not a dangerous condition, it can dramatically lower the self-esteem and confidence with individuals who suffer from it. Additionally, it can also result and produce significant scarring if an acne sufferer squeezes or otherwise irritates the affected portions of skin.

In particular, acne is the result of over-activity from the glands in our skin that produce oil and grease, in particular *sebum*. These glands and the sebum provide a useful function; they protect the skin, making it waterproof and reducing friction. Sebum also helps control our temperature, preventing us from getting too hot and slowing down the process of dehydration when we have not consumed enough water.

However, when these glands produce too much sebum, pores and hair follicles can become blocked, producing whiteheads and blackheads.

Furthermore, sebum is known to influence the behavior of *Propionbacterium acnes* often abbreviated to *P. acnes*. *P. acnes* is one of the many types of bacteria that flourish on the surface of human skin and which we usually do not notice or otherwise pay attention to. In fact, the presence of these bacteria is, in general, beneficial as they prevent harmful pathogens from surviving on our skin.

However, *P. acnes* feeds on the sebum our skin glands produce and thus during puberty and other conditions which cause excess sebum to be produced, *P. acnes* thrives and spreads. P. acnes produces enzymes and other chemicals as waste products, which do not normally affect us. However, in certain concentration these waste products can damage our skin, causing inflammation as well as the production of pus.

Fortunately, the wheat belly diet can even help reduce acne. Wheat, grains and the other problematic carbohydrates sources ruled out by the wheat belly diet can contribute to acne and intensify the condition. This is due to the effect of the problematic carbohydrates on our body's insulin levels.

Insulin is the chemical your body produces to transform carbohydrates into fat and alter your metabolism. When the consumption of certain carbohydrates causes your blood sugar to spike, the result is a rapid increase and release on insulin in your body; at least for healthy individuals who do not suffer from diabetes.

Yet insulin, at least in large levels, increases the body's production of sebum. As increased sebum levels result in greater levels and activity of *P. acnes*, high insulin levels has been increasingly associated with acne. As wheat, grains and several carbohydrate sources cause high insulin levels to arise, it can be deduced that these too influence the susceptibility and intensity of acne.

If you or someone you know is suffering from acne and wishes to alleviate their symptoms, suggest the wheat belly diet to them. There is no direct 'cure' to acne, however through religiously following the wheat belly diet, you can almost eliminate acne from your skin.

Cholesterol & High Blood Pressure

Blood pressure is the amount of force the circulating blood in the body exerts on the walls of the veins and arteries on the circulatory system. Blood pressure is generally categorized in three ways; low (hypotension), normal and high (hypertension). Both hypotension and hypertension can produce adverse effects on the body. Hypotension can cause episodes of dizziness as well as fainting and various heart disorders. If your blood pressure falls too low, you can enter a state of shock which can deprive the brain of important nutrients as well as oxygen supply (which is life threatening).

However, hypertension is more relevant to the wheat belly diet. When the pressure your blood exerts is too high, your blood has an abrasive effect on your arteries and heart. Ultimately, hypertension causes an array of maladies including heart failure, dementia and the failure of the kidneys.

The regular western diet can cause hypertension in a variety of ways. Firstly, consuming an excess of salt can raise the amount of water your blood retains. This results in your blood having a greater volume, but the same amount of space within the arteries, veins and heart (resulting in high pressure). Although not the only cause, high levels of salt are prevalent in many types of bread, wheat-based sauces and wheat products that the wheat belly diet recommends to avoid.

In addition to salt consumption, being overweight also causes high blood pressure. In overweight or obese people, the heart is required to beat harder in order to pump blood further to cover all the excess fat and mass overweight people carry. Owing to the heart beating harder, the blood itself is pushed harder and blood pressure is increased. As previously mentioned, wheat, grains and many other types of carbohydrates massively contribute to weight gain and obesity; therefore, by extension, these carbohydrates also often increase your blood pressure.

Furthermore, wheat, grains and the other carbohydrates mentioned also increase water retention (oedema). In a manner similar to excess salt intake, oedema increases the pressure of the blood resulting in hypertension. Naturally, as the wheat belly diet avoids the before mentioned problematic carbohydrates, oedema does not occur and blood pressure can become lower.

Unfortunately, cholesterol is also massively linked to blood pressure as well as associated dietary factor also linked with blood pressure.

Cholesterol is a type of essential fatty product your body makes which is important in the construction of multiple hormones as well as cell membranes and the production of vitamin D. However, in excess, cholesterol can be life threatening; cholesterol in the blood can cling to and clog up your arteries and veins (atherosclerosis), reducing the amount of room for your blood to flow. This not only results in hypertension (due to less space) but also heart attacks, blood clots and stroke.

However, the real clincher is that high cholesterol levels are partially *caused* by hypertension. As high pressure blood courses around your arteries, veins and heart it erodes the walls of these arteries and veins and these eroded walls are susceptible to cholesterol sticking to them and forming plaques, leading to atherosclerosis. Ultimately, there is a positive feedback loop between high blood pressure and high cholesterol; a feedback loop that can be broken through the wheat belly diet which can lower blood pressure.

Asthma & Breathing Problems

Asthma is a long term breathing disease caused by inflammation of the airways. Asthma can occasionally cause the airways to become blocked, which can be fatal, but more commonly causes coughing, wheezing as well shallowness of breath.

Asthma can severely impair one's ability to exercise as well as increase one's susceptibility and lower one's tolerance to airborne allergens such as dust or pollen.

The exact causes of asthma are not known; there are thought to be several genetic and environmental causes that contribute to the condition.

However, the wheat belly diet may be able to alleviate and reduce the causes and symptoms of asthma. As previously mentioned, asthma is ultimately a result of the inflammation of the airways, which in turn produces a range of other effects and symptoms (such as obstruction). It is known that the ingestion of wheat, in many people, causes inflammatory responses.

Wheat contains gliadins as well as many other genetic components related to grass and plant seeds that may cause the immune system to respond to a pathogenic threat, even if none exists.

Even if you or someone you know does not have diagnosed wheat allergies or wheat intolerance, it may be the wheat in their diet that is producing or worsening their asthma symptoms.

BLOATING & CONSTIPATION

Although not a frequent conversation topic, many people in the western world suffer from bloating or constipation.

Bloating is the sensation due to the swelling of the abdominal area, most notably the stomach. Bloating may cause this area to become excessively uncomfortable, or even painful. It can even result in shallowness of the breath as the diaphragm is obstructed by the swollen stomach and cannot contract and expand naturally.

Bloating can be caused by several diseases such as irritable bowel syndrome or even Crohn's disease, but it may also be due to poor functioning of the digestive system. Bloating is often the result of excess gas being produced in the stomach and small intestine, which in turn results from poor digestion of food. Likewise, bloating can also due to food being processed by the digestive system especially slowly with great difficulty.

This poor functioning of the stomach and small intestine, as you might have guessed by now, may be due to the wheat in your diet. The inflammatory and immune system responses associated with wheat also affect the stomach and immune system, which can prevent normal functioning of these areas. When the stomach and small intestine are influenced by inflammation due to the immune system, they cannot process the food you consume and hence you become bloated.

It is a similar story for constipation. Furthermore, constipation can also be caused by a lack of water in your digestive system, making it harder for matter to pass through the bowels. As previously mentioned, wheat and many other grains are responsible for excess water retention, which may be preventing the water in your body from being accessed where it needs to be; in your bowels therefore resulting in constipation.

Finally, wheat also damages the flora in your bowels. Although you may not be aware of the fact, within your small intestine live a huge variety of bacteria, most of which are harmless and help with the digestion and absorption of nutrients from food.

However, all the harmful molecules and substances within wheat such as gliadins upset the normal balance and levels of these bacteria within your bowels. Useful and harmless bacteria do not thrive on these substances, but dangerous and disruptive bacteria can thrive on them. This can result in your food not being digested and absorbed properly as well as various unnecessary waste products (such as excess gas). All of this can contribute and worsen bloating and constipation.

If you find yourself unhappy with your digestive system, try the wheat belly diet; you are bound to find yourself spending less time thinking about your bowels and more time enjoying your life.

MIGRAINE RELIEF

A migraine is a type of extreme headache, usually experienced as a painful pulsing sensation from the head. Additionally, many people experience additional symptoms such as heightened experience or visual or auditory stimulus (usually to the extent which these stimuli become painful or unpleasant).

The causes of migraines are not yet understood. Migraines often tend to run in the family, suggesting that genetic factors may be influential. Others have suggested migraines are the result of transient changes to the neuro-chemical balance of the brain and changes to the brain's blood flow.

However, many people who embrace the wheat belly diet for it's other benefits are also realizing the positive impacts of this diet on migraine frequency and intensity. Although the relationship between the wheat belly diet and relief of migraine symptoms has not been scientifically explored, the evidence from wheat belly dieters is ever-increasing. If you suffer from painful migraines and cannot find sanctuary with medicine (or reject the constant need for painkillers) try the wheat belly diet and follow the footsteps of many other migraine sufferers.

BRAIN FOG

It is not uncommon for westerners to suffer from an elusive and hard to describe 'brain fog'. 'Brain fog refers to a difficulty in thinking with lucidity and a lack of effort. Too many individuals, even if they can function 'normally', feel as if they cannot concentrate. There is something causing an innate resistance and difficulty when trying to think, often with significant psychological and emotional impacts. It is hard to enjoy life with zest and vigor if your brain is constantly struggling to keep up with your life.

However, brain fog may be caused due to a poor diet. In particular, inability to concentrate and a lack of mental energy may be the result of an excess of carbohydrate in the diet and a lack of fats. The human brain is predominantly fatty tissue and requires a constant supply of fatty acids to perform optimally, such as omega-3 fatty acids and DHA. A diet where the majority of calories come from wheat, grains and other carbohydrates may struggle to provide enough of these fatty acids for the brain to thrive, potentially causing 'brain fog'.

The wheat belly diet is one solution to the brain fog dilemma; the diet advocates multiple sources of essential fatty acids, which are the key to good brain health – nuts, seeds, oils and fish. If you find that your brain will simply not allow your mind to work properly, try the wheat belly diet; it has worked for others and it can work for you!

CONCLUSION

Maintaining a good diet is essential for well being and happiness. In our vanity, almost all the emphasis in the western world is on weight loss and looking slim and fit. Although avoiding obesity and excess weight is essential for good health, there is much more to having a healthy diet and lifestyle than being thin.

Far too many individuals, although petit and slender, suffer physiologically and psychologically because their diet is poor. It may be the case that they do not get enough fats in their diet or that they suffer from allergic responses to the foods they eat, or a myriad of other symptoms. The worse aspect of these dietary failures is how under-appreciated and poorly recognized they are; almost everyone fails to properly attribute a variety of ailments to poor diet, often citing vague and non-responsible factors such as stress or depression for their problems.

This book has provided you with insight into how the wheat belly diet can possibly cure 10 of the most common health ailments in western society. From blood pressure and cholesterol, to acne and aging. The benefits of the wheat belly diet are widespread and vast.

Even if you are fortunate to not suffer from these conditions presently, if you continue to gorge yourself on the poor average western diet, these problems will surely manifest. No matter your current level of well being, take an interest in your health and body today and transition to the wheat belly diet; it is guaranteed to improve your happiness and well being in the long-term.

ABOUT THE AUTHOR

I am a mother to three beautiful children and a wife to a wonderful husband. I have a passion to teach others and can often be found volunteering in my local community.

During college I worked within my family catering business to support myself. After graduating I opened a chain of small cafes that I ran successfully for a number of years. Now whilst being a stay at home mom, I am able share my skills, knowledge and experience through my books. I feel a great deal of satisfaction when helping others and seeing them flourish to their maximum potential.

Please check out my author page on Amazon to see my latest publications. Please don't forget to join my Book Club for a free books, newsletters and updates.

Once again I want to thank you for reading my book. I really hope you got a lot out of it.

If you enjoyed this book I would really appreciate it if you could leave me a positive review on Amazon. You can **click here** to go directly to the book on Amazon and leave your review.

I love getting feedback from my readers and reviews on Amazon really do make a difference. I read all my reviews and would really appreciate your thoughts.

Thanks so much.

CHARLOTTE MOYER

OTHER BOOKS BY AUTHOR

WHEAT BELLY: 21 DAY WHEAT-FREE PLAN, FULL OF QUICK & NUTRITIOUS RECIPES

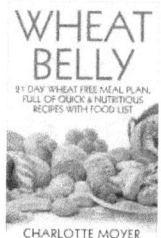

WHEAT BELLY: 31 DELICIOUS WHEAT FREE RECIPES TO LOSE WEIGHT FAST

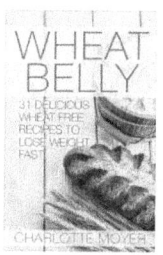

VEGAN: 35 HIGH PROTEIN VEGAN RECIPES FOR WEIGHT LOSS AND BUILDING MUSCLE

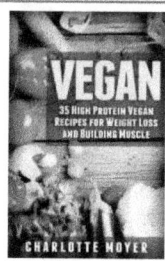

How to Bake Perfectly: 101 Tips, Tricks & Cheats for Baking Recipes

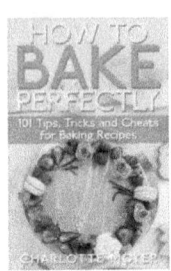

How to Make Money from Home: 7 Steps to Make Money from Baking recipes

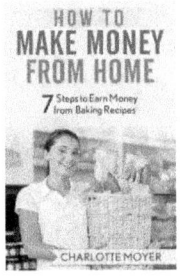

www.ingramcontent.com/pod-product-compliance
Lightning Source LLC
Chambersburg PA
CBHW072019290526
45787CB00013B/1342